FRAGRANCE OILS FOR HOME DECOR:

ENHANCING YOUR LIVING SPACE WITH SCENT

E. O. COFFIE

Fragrance Oils for Home Décor: Enhancing Your Living Space with Scent

Fragrance Oils for Home Décor: Enhancing Your Living Space with Scent

@ 2023 Elizabeth Coffie

Published by The Adonaifields Group of Companies
and imprint of ECM Elizabeth Coffie Media
First Edition - April 2023.
Visit our website: www.eoocsoapsandoils.com
All rights reserved.

No part of this publication may be reproduced, stored in a retrieval system, or be transmitted, in any form, or by any means, mechanical, electronic, photocopying or otherwise without prior written consent of the publisher.

Fragrance Oils for Home Décor: Enhancing Your Living Space with Scent

Table Of Contents

Fragrance Oils for Home Décor: Enhancing Your Living Space with Scent

Fragrance Oils for Home Décor: Enhancing Your Living Space with Scent

Introduction

Welcome and explanation of the purpose of the book

Welcome to "Fragrance Oils for Home Décor: Enhancing Your Living Space with Scent"! This book has been written with you, the retail end user, in mind. Whether you are a seasoned aromatherapy enthusiast or a newcomer to the world of fragrance oils, this book will provide you with valuable insights into how you can use these oils to enhance your living space and create a more inviting atmosphere in your home.

The purpose of this book is twofold. Firstly, we aim to provide you with a comprehensive overview of the different types of fragrance oils that are available on the market, their properties, and how they can be used to enhance your home décor. From floral and fruity scents to earthy and woody aromas, there is a fragrance oil out there to suit every taste and preference.

Secondly, we want to show you how you can use fragrance oils to create a more relaxing and soothing atmosphere in your home.

Fragrance Oils for Home Décor: Enhancing Your Living Space with Scent

Whether you are looking to reduce stress, enhance your mood, or simply create a more pleasant environment, fragrance oils can help you achieve your goals.

Throughout this book, you will find practical tips and advice on how to select the right fragrance oils for your home décor needs, as well as step-by-step instructions on how to use them effectively. We will also provide you with information on the different types of diffusers that are available on the market, so that you can choose the right one for your needs and preferences.

In conclusion, "Fragrance Oils for Home Décor: Enhancing Your Living Space with Scent" is a must-read for anyone who is interested in aromatherapy essential and fragrance oils. We hope that this book will inspire you to explore the world of fragrance oils and discover the many benefits that they can bring to your home and your life.

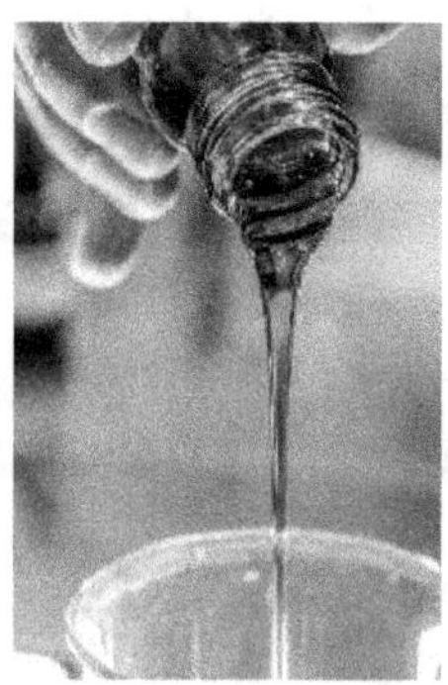

Fragrance Oils for Home Décor: Enhancing Your Living Space with Scent

Brief history of fragrance oils and their uses in home décor

Fragrance oils have been in use for centuries in various cultures around the world. The earliest records of fragrance use date back to ancient Egypt, where aromatic oils were used for religious and cosmetic purposes. The Greeks and Romans also used fragrances extensively, both as perfumes and in their homes.

In medieval Europe, fragrance oils were used primarily in the form of incense. They were burned in churches and homes to create a pleasant atmosphere and mask unpleasant odors. During the Renaissance period, the use of fragrance oils became more popular, and they were used in a variety of ways. They were mixed with wax to create scented candles, used in potpourri, and added to bathwater for a relaxing experience.

Aromatherapy essential and fragrance oils are especially popular in home décor. Aromatherapy has been used for centuries as a natural way to promote relaxation, reduce stress, and improve overall well-being. Essential oils are extracted from plants and are used for their therapeutic properties. Fragrance oils are synthetic and are used primarily for their scent.

Fragrance Oils for Home Décor: Enhancing Your Living Space with Scent

In modern times, fragrance oils have become even more popular, and their uses have expanded to include home décor. They are used in diffusers, candles, and air fresheners to create a pleasant scent in any room. Fragrance oils are also used in cleaning products, laundry detergents, and personal care items such as lotions and soaps.

There are many different fragrance oils available, each with its own unique scent and properties. Some popular scents include lavender, peppermint, and eucalyptus. Lavender is known for its calming properties and is often used in diffusers and candles to promote relaxation. Peppermint is invigorating and is often used in air fresheners and cleaning products. Eucalyptus is known for its ability to clear the sinuses and is often used in diffusers and bath products.

Fragrance oils have a long and fascinating history, and their uses in home décor have expanded greatly over the years.

Whether you are looking to create a relaxing atmosphere in your home or simply add a pleasant scent to a room, fragrance oils are a versatile and effective way to enhance your living space with scent.

Explanation of the benefits of using fragrance oils in home décor

Fragrance oils are becoming increasingly popular in the world of home décor as people are discovering the benefits of using them to enhance the ambiance of their living spaces. Unlike essential oils, fragrance oils are synthetic and are designed to mimic the scents of natural substances such as fruits, flowers, and herbs.

These oils are often used in candles, diffusers, and potpourri to create an inviting and relaxing environment. In this subchapter, we will explore the benefits of using fragrance oils in home décor.

Firstly, fragrance oils are an affordable and convenient way to add fragrance to your home. Unlike essential oils, which can be expensive and difficult to find, fragrance oils are widely available and come in a variety of scents. This means that you can easily find a fragrance oil that suits your taste and budget.

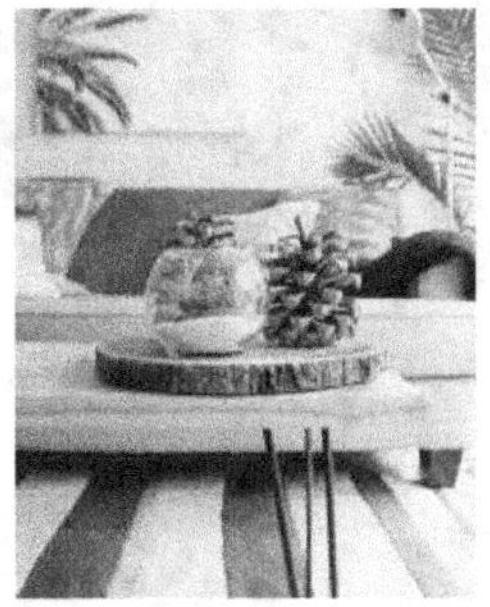

Fragrance Oils for Home Décor: Enhancing Your Living Space with Scent

Secondly, fragrance oils are long-lasting and can provide a continuous scent for hours. This makes them perfect for use in rooms that are frequently occupied, such as the living room or bedroom. Additionally, fragrance oils can be used in a variety of ways, such as in diffusers, candles, and wax melts, giving you the flexibility to choose the best method for your living space.

Thirdly, fragrance oils can be used to create a specific mood or atmosphere in your home. For example, lavender fragrance oil can be used to promote relaxation and calmness, while citrus scents can help to energize and uplift your mood. This makes fragrance oils perfect for use in aromatherapy and can be a great addition to your self-care routine.

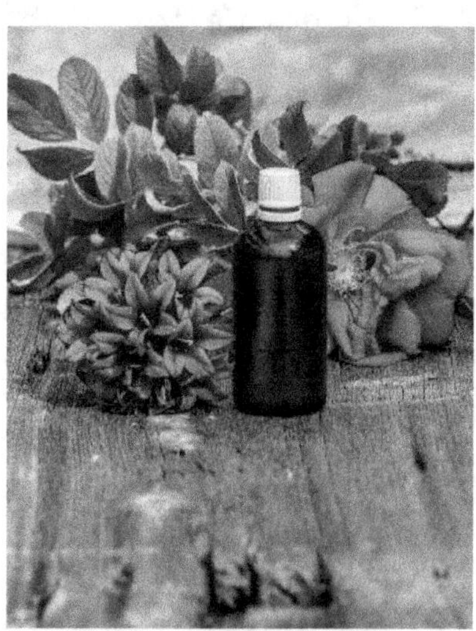

Fragrance Oils for Home Décor: Enhancing Your Living Space with Scent

Lastly, fragrance oils can be used to mask unpleasant odors in your home. If you have pets or live in a busy area, you may find that your living space has unpleasant smells. Fragrance oils can help to eliminate these odors and replace them with a pleasant scent.

Fragrance oils are a versatile and affordable way to enhance the ambiance of your living space. Whether you are looking to create a relaxing atmosphere or mask unpleasant odors, fragrance oils offer a range of benefits that make them a great addition to your home.

Understanding Fragrance Oils

Definition and explanation of fragrance oils

Fragrance oils are a popular way to add scent to your home or office. They are often used in aromatherapy and home décor, and are available in a wide variety of scents. In this chapter, we will define and explain fragrance oils, including how they are made and how they can be used.

Definition of Fragrance Oils:

Fragrance oils are often used in candles, diffusers, and other home décor items, as well as in personal care products such as perfumes and lotions.

Fragrance oils can be made from a wide variety of ingredients, including essential oils, synthetic compounds, and natural extracts. However,essential oils are typically created through a process of distillation or extraction, which involves extracting the scent compounds from plant material or other sources.

Fragrance Oils for Home Décor: Enhancing Your Living Space with Scent

Explanation of Fragrance Oils

Fragrance oils are often used in aromatherapy, which is the practice of using scents to promote physical and emotional well-being. Aromatherapy essential and fragrance oils can be used in a variety of ways, including in baths, or in massage oils.

When using fragrance oils in aromatherapy, it is important to choose scents that are appropriate for the intended effect. For example, lavender is often used to promote relaxation, while peppermint can be invigorating and energizing.

Fragrance oils can also be used to add scent to a room. They are often used in candles or diffusers, which release the scent into the air. When choosing fragrance oils for home décor, it is important to consider the overall aesthetic of the room and choose a scent that complements it.

Fragrance oils are a versatile and popular way to add scent to your personal care products, and are available in a wide variety of scents. When choosing fragrance oils, it is important to consider the intended effect and the overall aesthetic of the space.

Differences between essential oils and fragrance oils

When it comes to scenting your home, there are two main types of oils you can use – essential oils and fragrance oils. While both can provide a pleasant aroma, there are some significant differences between the two.

Essential oils are extracted from plants through a distillation process. They contain the natural scent and essence of the plant and can offer a range of therapeutic benefits when used in aromatherapy. Essential oils are often used in diffusers or added to carrier oils for use in massage or skincare products.

On the other hand, fragrance oils are synthetic or artificial oils that are created to mimic a specific scent. They are typically used in candles, soaps, and other home fragrance products. Because they are not derived from natural sources, they do not offer the same therapeutic benefits as essential oils.

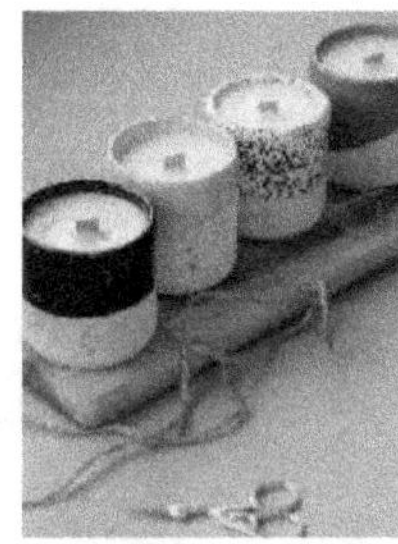

Fragrance Oils for Home Décor: Enhancing Your Living Space with Scent

One of the main differences between essential oils and fragrance oils is their purity. Essential oils are pure and natural, while fragrance oils are a blend of synthetic chemicals. Essential oils are also more potent than fragrance oils, which means you need less of them to achieve a strong scent. This is because essential oils are concentrated and can be quite strong on their own.

Another difference is their longevity. Fragrance oils tend to have a longer shelf life than essential oils, which can degrade over time. This means that your essential oil products may not smell as strong after a few months, while your fragrance oil products can last for years if stored properly. This is because fragrance oils are manufactured.

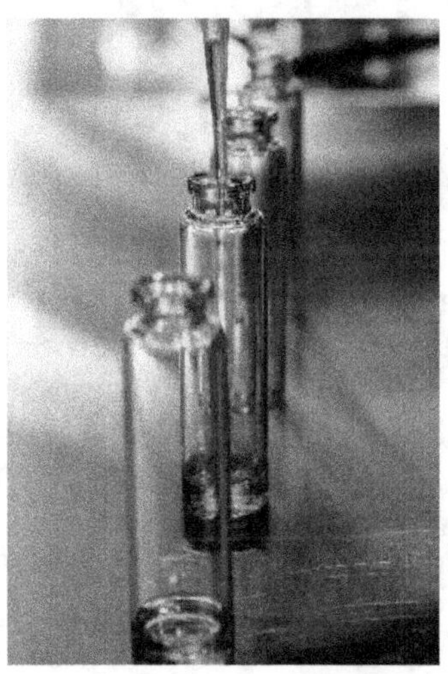

Fragrance Oils for Home Décor: Enhancing Your Living Space with Scent

Lastly, essential oils are often more expensive than fragrance oils. This is because they are extracted from natural sources and require a significant amount of plant material to produce a small amount of oil. Fragrance oils, on the other hand, are created in a lab and are much cheaper to produce.

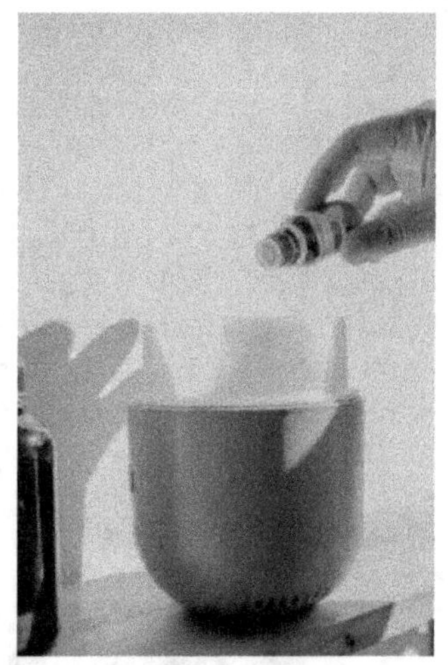

In summary, while both essential oils and fragrance oils can provide a pleasant aroma, there are some significant differences between the two. Essential oils are natural, pure, and offer therapeutic benefits, while fragrance oils are synthetic and are used for their scent. When choosing oils for your home décor, consider these differences and choose the option that best fits your needs and preferences.

Understanding the composition of fragrance oils

Understanding the Composition of Fragrance Oils

Fragrance oils have become increasingly popular in recent years, with more and more people using them to enhance the ambiance of their homes. Whether you're using them for aromatherapy, to create a relaxing atmosphere, or simply to add a pleasant scent to your living space, it's important to understand the composition of fragrance oils.

Fragrance oils are made up of a combination of natural and synthetic ingredients. The exact composition can vary depending on the brand and the specific scent, but there are some common components you'll find in most fragrance oils.

The first component is the base oil. This is usually a carrier oil like jojoba or almond oil, which is used to dilute the fragrance and make it safe to use on the skin or in a diffuser. The base oil also helps to carry the scent and make it last longer.

Fragrance Oils for Home Décor: Enhancing Your Living Space with Scent

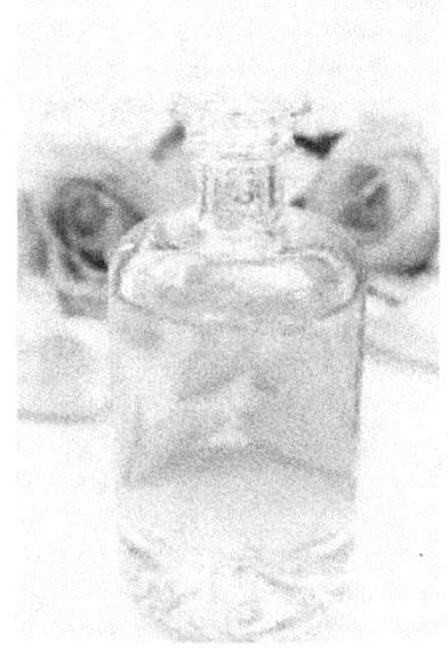

The second component is the fragrance itself. This can be a combination of natural and synthetic ingredients, which work together to create a specific scent. Natural ingredients like essential oils are often used to create the top notes of a fragrance, while synthetic ingredients are used to create the base notes.

The third component is the fixative. This is an ingredient that helps to hold the fragrance together and make it last longer. Common fixatives include musk, amber, and vanilla.

When choosing a fragrance oil, it's important to look at the ingredients list and choose a brand that uses high-quality, natural ingredients. Pure synthetic fragrances can be harsh and irritating to the skin if not dilluted or used properly.

Fragrance Oils for Home Décor: Enhancing Your Living Space with Scent

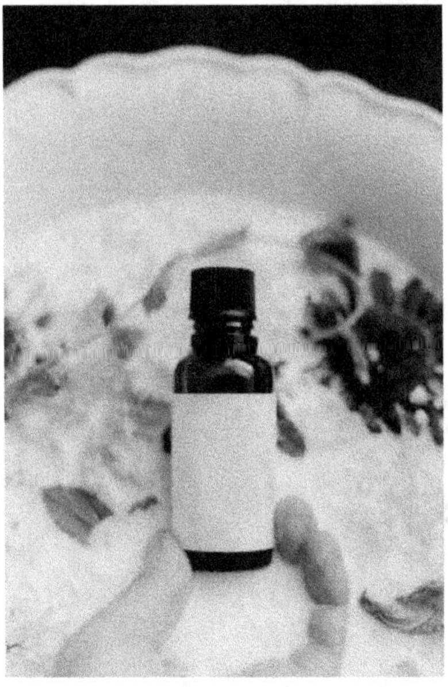

It's also important to consider the concentration of the fragrance oil. A higher concentration will give you a stronger scent, but it may also be more expensive. If you're using the fragrance oil in a diffuser, a lower concentration may be more appropriate.

Understanding the composition of fragrance oils is key to choosing the right product for your needs. Look for high-quality, natural ingredients and consider the concentration of the fragrance oil to get the best results. With the right fragrance oil, you can enhance the ambiance of your home and create a relaxing, inviting atmosphere.

Fragrance Oils for Home Décor: Enhancing Your Living Space with Scent

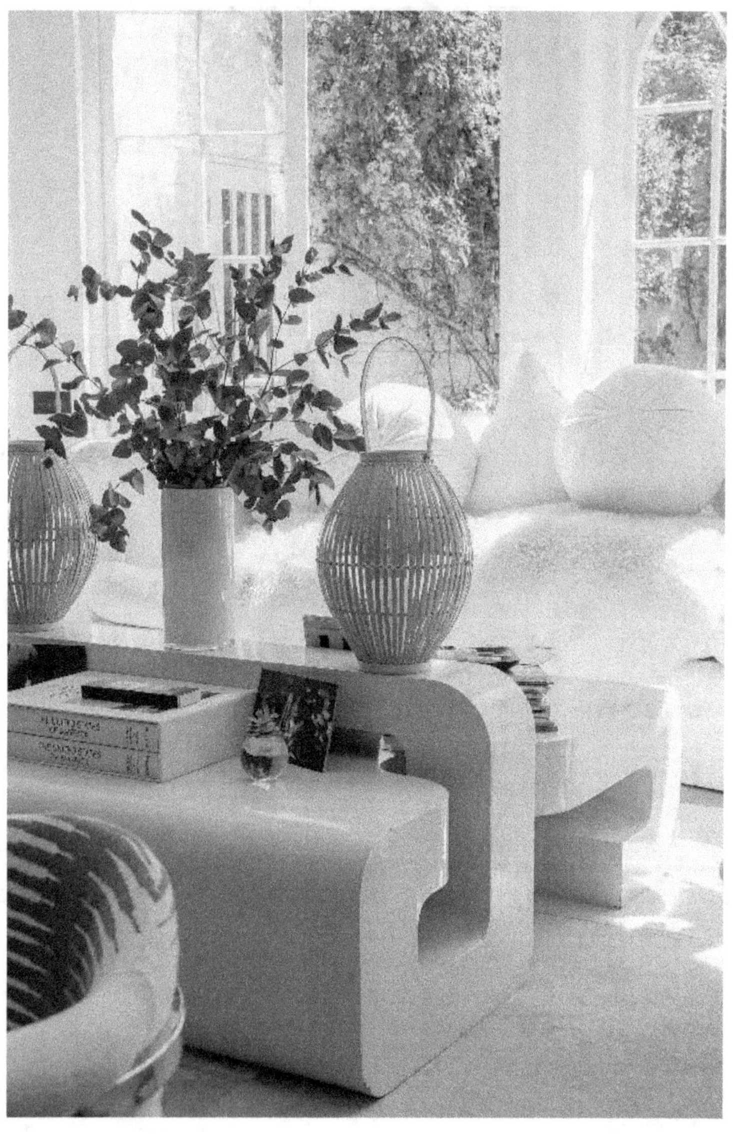

Fragrance Oils for Home Décor: Enhancing Your Living Space with Scent

How to choose the right fragrance oil for your home décor

Fragrance oils are a popular choice for those who love to enhance their living space with aroma. They are versatile, affordable, and easy to use. However, choosing the right fragrance oil can be overwhelming, especially if you are new to this world of scents. In this subchapter, we will discuss some tips on how to choose the right fragrance oil for your home décor.

1. Consider the Purpose

Before choosing a fragrance oil, consider what you want to achieve with it. Are you looking for a relaxing scent to use in your bedroom? Or a refreshing scent to use in your living room? Different fragrances have different effects on our mood and emotions.

2. Choose the Right Type of Fragrance Oil

Fragrance oils come in different types, such as essential oils, fragrance oils, and blended oils. The difference is that essential oils are natural oils extracted from plants, while fragrance oils are synthetic oils that mimic the scent of natural ingredients.

Fragrance Oils for Home Décor: Enhancing Your Living Space with Scent

Blended oils are a combination of essential and fragrance oils. Each type has its own benefits and drawbacks, so choose the one that suits your preferences.

3. Check the Concentration

Fragrance oils come in different concentration levels, ranging from 1% to 100%. The higher the concentration, the stronger the scent. However, a high concentration may not always be suitable for your needs. For example, if you have a small room, a high concentration of fragrance oil may be overpowering. On the other hand, if you have a large room, a low concentration may not be noticeable enough.

4. Test the Fragrance

Before purchasing a fragrance oil, test it to see how it smells in your home. You can do this by using a fragrance oil diffuser or by placing a few drops on a cotton ball and placing it in the room. This will give you an idea of how the scent will interact with your home décor and whether it is suitable for your needs.

In conclusion, choosing the right fragrance oil for your home décor requires some consideration and experimentation. By following these tips, you can find the perfect scent to enhance your living space and create a welcoming and relaxing environment.

How to Use Fragrance Oils for Home Décor

Different ways to use fragrance oils in home décor

Fragrance oils are not just used for perfumes and body oils; they can also be used as a decorative element in home décor. There are many different ways to incorporate fragrance oils into your living space, and the possibilities are endless. In this subchapter, we will explore some of the most popular ways to use fragrance oils in home décor.

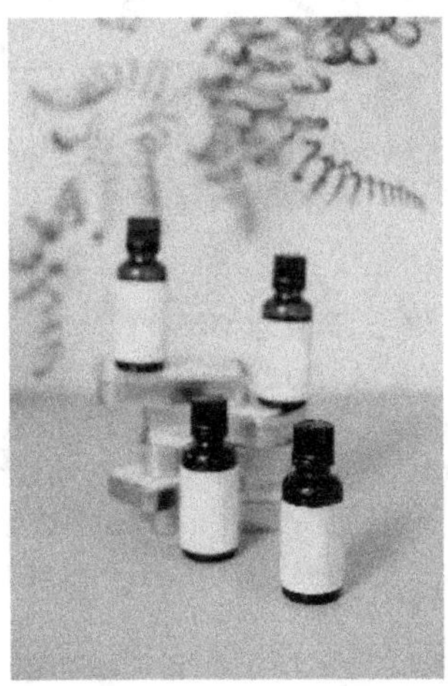

Fragrance Oils for Home Décor: Enhancing Your Living Space with Scent

1. Diffusers
One of the most common ways to use fragrance oils in home décor is through the use of diffusers. Diffusers come in a variety of styles and designs and can be placed in any room of your home. They work by releasing the fragrance oil into the air, filling your living space with a pleasant aroma.

2. Potpourri
Potpourri is another popular way to use fragrance oils in home décor. You can create your own potpourri by mixing dried flowers, leaves, and other natural elements with fragrance oils. This can be placed in a decorative bowl or sachet and placed in any room of your home.

3. Candles
Candles are a classic way to add fragrance to your home décor. They come in a variety of scents and styles and can be used in any room of your home. You can also create your own candles by adding fragrance oils to melted wax and pouring it into a mold.

4. Room Sprays
Room sprays are another effective way to use fragrance oils in home décor. They work by spraying a fragrant mist into the air, filling your living space with a pleasant aroma. Room sprays come in a variety of scents and can be used in any room of your home.

Fragrance Oils for Home Décor: Enhancing Your Living Space with Scent

5. Linens

Fragrance oils can also be used to add fragrance to your linens. You can add a few drops of fragrance oil to your laundry detergent or fabric softener to infuse your clothes and linens with a pleasant scent. You can also create your own linen spray by mixing fragrance oil with water and spraying it onto your linens.

Fragrance oils can be a great addition to your home décor. They can be used in a variety of ways and can add a pleasant aroma to your living space. Whether you choose to use fragrance oils in diffusers, potpourri, candles, room sprays, or linens, the possibilities are endless. So go ahead and experiment with different scents and find the perfect fragrance oil to enhance your living space.

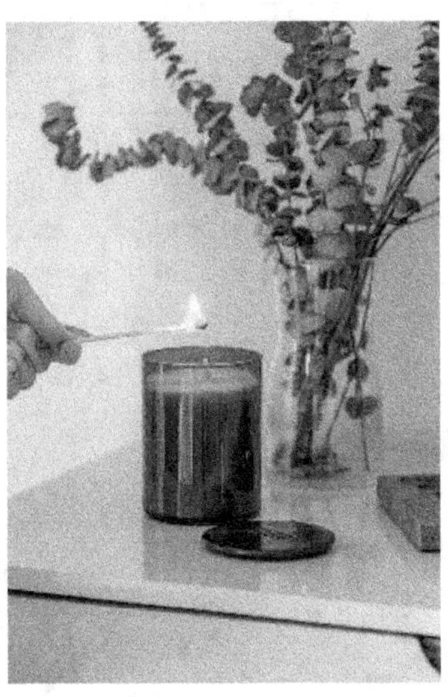

How to make fragrance oil diffusers

Fragrance oil diffusers are a great addition to any home décor. They not only add a pleasant fragrance to the room but also have therapeutic benefits. Making your own fragrance oil diffuser is a fun and easy DIY project that you can do at home. Here's how to make fragrance oil diffusers:

Materials Needed:

- Glass container with a narrow opening
- Fibre/Rattan reeds or bamboo skewers
- Diffuser Base or Carrier oil such as sweet almond oil, fractionated coconut oil or jojoba oil
- Essential oils or fragrance oils of your choice
- Funnel

Instructions:

Step 1: Choose a glass container with a narrow opening. The narrow opening will help slow down the evaporation of the oil, making your diffuser last longer.

Step 2: Pour your diffuser base or if you prefer to use a carrier oil into the glass container. Diffuser bases or carrier oils help to dilute the essential or fragrance oils and helps them diffuse slowly.

Fragrance Oils for Home Décor: Enhancing Your Living Space with Scent

Step 3: Add your essential oils or fragrance oils. You can use a single essential or fragrance oil or mix and match to create your own unique blend. The recommended ratio is 20-25 drops of oil per 1/4 cup of carrier oil.

Step 4: Mix the base or fragrance oils and carrier oil together using a funnel.

Step 5: Insert the fibre/rattan reeds or bamboo skewers into the glass container. Allow the reeds or skewers to soak up the oil mixture for a few hours before flipping them over.

Step 6: Flip the reeds or skewers over every few days to refresh the scent.

Step 7: Enjoy your homemade fragrance oil diffuser!

Tips:

- Use high-quality carrier oils and essential or fragrance oils for best results.
- Experiment with different oils and blends to find your favorite scent.
- Consider the size of the room when choosing the number of reeds or skewers to use. The larger the room, the more reeds or skewers you will need.

Fragrance Oils for Home Décor: Enhancing Your Living Space with Scent

Making your own fragrance oil diffuser is a simple and cost-effective way to add a pleasant scent to your home while also enjoying the therapeutic benefits of essential oils. With a few simple steps, you can create your own unique blend and enjoy the benefits of aromatherapy in your own space.

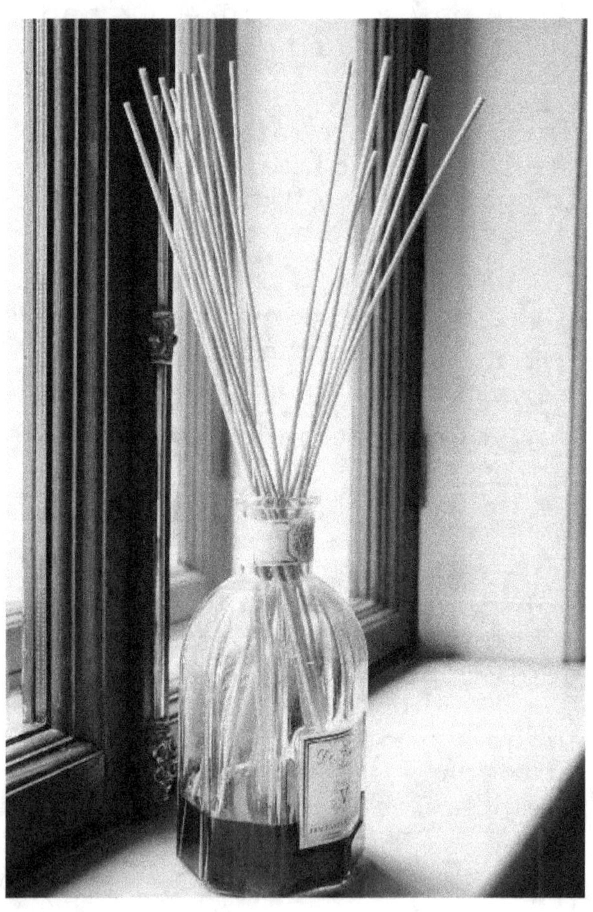

Fragrance Oils for Home Décor: Enhancing Your Living Space with Scent

How to make room sprays

Room sprays are an excellent way to add a touch of fragrance to your home. They are easy to make, and you can customize them to suit your preferences. In this section, we will discuss how to make room sprays using fragrance oils.

To make a room spray, you will need a few basic ingredients. You will need a spray bottle, distilled water, and fragrance oil. You can find all of these items at your local craft store or online.

To start, fill the spray bottle with distilled water. You can use tap water, but the minerals in the water can affect the scent of the room spray. Then, add a few drops of fragrance oil to the water. The number of drops you use will depend on the strength of the fragrance oil and the size of the spray bottle. We recommend using no more than 10-15 drops per 8 oz spray bottle.

Once you have added the fragrance oil, shake the bottle to mix the ingredients. You can test the scent by spraying a small amount in the air and smelling it. If you find the scent too weak, you can add a few more drops of fragrance oil. If the scent is too strong, you can dilute the mixture with more distilled water.

Fragrance Oils for Home Décor: Enhancing Your Living Space with Scent

When you are satisfied with the scent, label the spray bottle with the fragrance name and the date you made it. This will help you keep track of the different scents you have made.

To use the room spray, simply shake the bottle and spray it in the air. You can also spray it on fabrics, such as curtains or pillows, to add a touch of fragrance to the room.

Making room sprays is a simple and fun way to enhance the scent of your home. By using fragrance oils, you can customize the scents to suit your preferences and create a unique atmosphere in your living space.

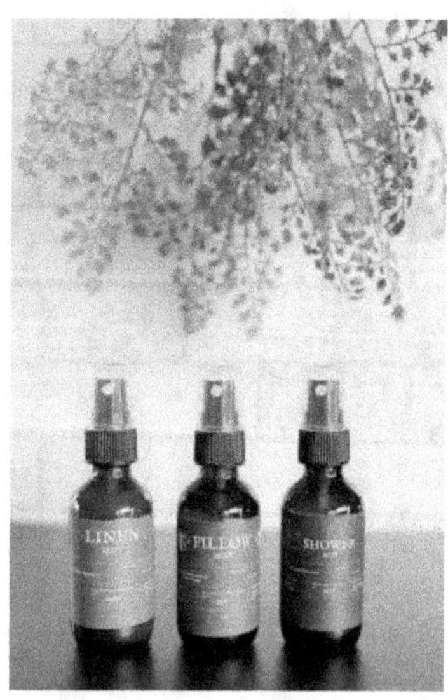

Fragrance Oils for Home Décor: Enhancing Your Living Space with Scent

How to make potpourri

Potpourri is a great way to add fragrance to your home without using candles or diffusers. It is a mixture of dried flowers, herbs, and spices, and can be customized to your liking. Making your own potpourri is easy and fun, and can be a great way to get kids involved in crafting.

To make potpourri, you will need:

- Dried flowers and herbs
- Spices and essential oils
- A container with a lid
- A spoon for mixing

First, choose your dried flowers and herbs. You can use any combination of flowers and herbs that you like, but make sure they are completely dry before using them. Some popular options include lavender, rose petals, and chamomile.

Next, add some spices and essential oils to your mixture. This is where you can really customize your potpourri to your liking. Some popular spices include cinnamon, cloves, and nutmeg. You can also add essential oils for an extra burst of fragrance. Some good options include lavender, peppermint, and lemon.

Fragrance Oils for Home Décor: Enhancing Your Living Space with Scent

Mix everything together in a container with a lid. You can use a Mason jar or any other type of container that has a tight-fitting lid. Make sure everything is mixed together well, and then let the potpourri sit for a few days to let the fragrance develop.

Once your potpourri is ready, you can display it in a decorative dish or jar in any room of your home. You can also put it in a sachet and tuck it in your drawers or closets to keep your clothes smelling fresh.

Making your own potpourri is a great way to experiment with different fragrances and create a unique scent for your home. It is also a great way to use up any flowers or herbs that you may have left over from other projects. So why not try making some potpourri today and see how it can enhance your home décor?

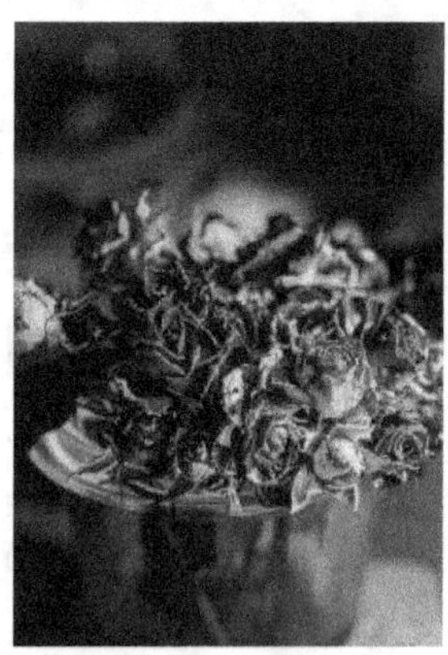

How to make scented candles

Scented candles are a delightful addition to any home, and they provide a relaxing and calming atmosphere. Making your scented candles is a fun and easy process that you can enjoy with your friends and family. In this chapter, we will guide you through the steps to make scented candles using fragrance oils.

To make scented candles, you will need:

- Wax (soy wax is an excellent option)
- Wicks
- Fragrance oil
- Color blocks or dye (don't use water dye)
- Heat-resistant containers
- Thermometer
- Double boiler or a pot and a heatproof bowl
- Stirring utensil

Step 1: Melt the wax

Begin by melting the soy wax in a double boiler or a pot and a heatproof bowl. Heat the wax until it reaches a temperature of 160°F, and then remove it from the heat source.

Step 2: Add color (optional)

Fragrance Oils for Home Décor: Enhancing Your Living Space with Scent

If you want to add color to your candles, now is the time to do so. You can use color blocks or dye to achieve your desired color. Remember to stir the mixture well to ensure the color is evenly distributed.

Step 3: Add the fragrance oil

Once the wax has cooled down to a temperature of 140°F, add the fragrance oil. The recommended amount of fragrance oil is 1 oz. per pound of wax, but you can adjust it to your preference. Don't add fragrance at any temperature higher than 140°F as if you do, the fragrance will evaporate. Stir the mixture thoroughly to ensure the fragrance oil is evenly distributed.

Step 4: Prepare the container

While waiting for the wax to cool down to 120°F the pouring temperature, prepare the container by securing the wick in the center of the container. You can use a wick sticker or hot glue to hold the wick in place.

Step 5: Pour the wax

Once the wax has cooled down to 120°F, it is time to pour it into the container.

Fragrance Oils for Home Décor: Enhancing Your Living Space with Scent

Slowly pour the wax into the container, making sure the wick stays in the center. Leave the candles to cool down and harden for at least 24 hours.

And there you have it – your very own scented candles! Making scented candles using fragrance oils is a fun and easy process that you can enjoy in the comfort of your home. Experiment with different fragrances and colors to create your unique candles that will enhance your living space with scent.

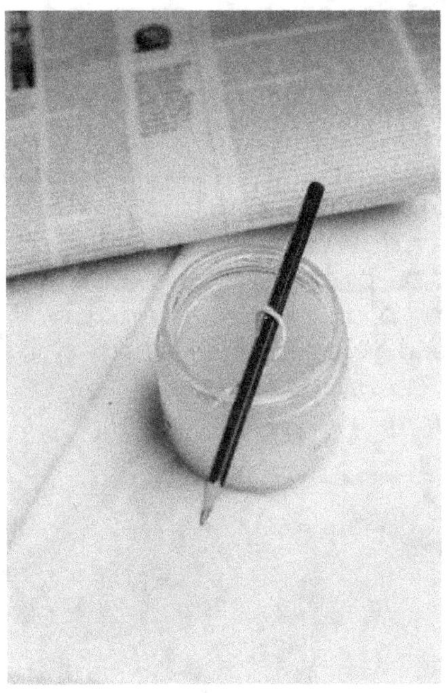

Popular Fragrance Oils for Home Décor

Lavender

Lavender is one of the most popular and versatile fragrances used in aromatherapy and home décor. Its scent is soothing, calming, and relaxing, making it ideal for a variety of applications. In this subchapter, we'll explore the benefits of lavender essential oil and how you can use it to enhance your living space with scent.

Lavender essential oil is derived from the flowers of the lavender plant. It has a light, floral scent that is both calming and refreshing. It is commonly used in aromatherapy to promote relaxation, reduce stress, and improve sleep quality. Lavender oil has also been shown to have antibacterial and anti-inflammatory properties, making it useful for treating skin conditions and minor injuries.

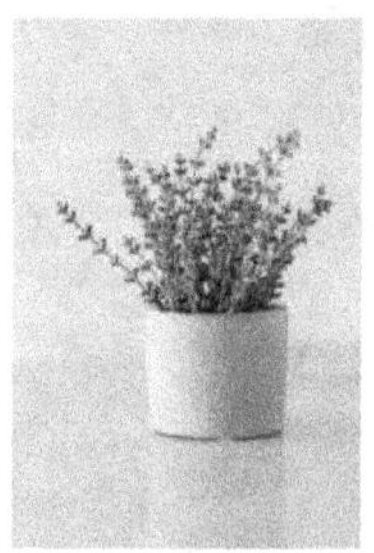

Fragrance Oils for Home Décor: Enhancing Your Living Space with Scent

One of the easiest ways to incorporate lavender into your home décor is through the use of candles or diffusers. A lavender-scented candle can create a calming atmosphere in any room, while a diffuser can release the scent of lavender throughout your home. You can also add a few drops of lavender essential oil to your laundry detergent or fabric softener to infuse your linens with the relaxing scent of lavender.

Another way to use lavender in your home is through the use of dried lavender flowers. These can be used in sachets or potpourri to add a subtle lavender scent to your drawers or closets. You can also use dried lavender to make your own lavender oil, which can be used in a variety of DIY projects such as bath salts, body scrubs, and massage oils.

In addition to its use in home décor, lavender essential oil is also commonly used in personal care products such as lotions, soaps, and shampoos. Its soothing properties make it ideal for use in products designed to promote relaxation and reduce stress.

Overall, lavender is a versatile and beneficial fragrance that can enhance your living space with its soothing and calming properties. Whether you choose to use it in candles, diffusers, or personal care products, lavender essential oil is a must-have for any aromatherapy or home décor enthusiast.

Peppermint

Peppermint oil is a popular fragrance oil that is widely used for its refreshing, invigorating, and uplifting aroma. It is extracted from the leaves of the peppermint plant, which is native to Europe and Asia but is now widely cultivated in many parts of the world.

Peppermint oil is known for its antiseptic, antifungal, and anti-inflammatory properties, making it a popular choice for aromatherapy, home remedies, and beauty products. It is also used in the food and beverage industry as a flavoring agent for confectionery, chewing gum, and other products.

In aromatherapy, peppermint oil is used to relieve stress, anxiety, and fatigue, as well as to improve mental clarity and concentration. It is also effective in relieving headaches, migraines, and sinus congestion. Peppermint oil can be used alone or in combination with other oils such as lavender, eucalyptus, and lemon.

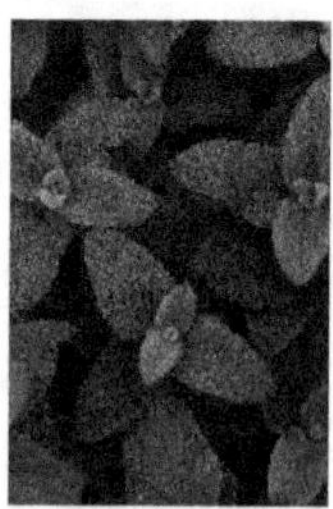

Fragrance Oils for Home Décor: Enhancing Your Living Space with Scent

Peppermint oil can also be used in home décor to create a refreshing and energizing atmosphere. It can be added to diffusers, potpourri, candles, and other décor items to infuse the space with its invigorating aroma. Peppermint oil can also be added to cleaning solutions and air fresheners to provide a natural and refreshing scent.

When using peppermint oil, it is important to dilute it properly to avoid skin irritation or other adverse reactions. It should also be kept out of reach of children and pets, as it can be toxic when ingested in large quantities.

Peppermint oil is a versatile fragrance oil that can be used for its aroma, therapeutic properties, and flavoring. It is a popular choice for aromatherapy, home décor, and personal care products, and is a must-have for anyone who wants to create a refreshing and energizing atmosphere in their living space.

Eucalyptus

Eucalyptus is a popular fragrance oil in the world of aromatherapy and home décor. Known for its refreshing and invigorating scent, eucalyptus is a versatile oil that can enhance the ambiance of any living space.

Extracted from the leaves of the eucalyptus tree, this essential oil has a strong, minty aroma that is both cooling and energizing. It is often used in diffusers, candles, and room sprays to promote relaxation, relieve stress, and clear the mind.

One of the most popular uses of eucalyptus oil is in the shower or bath. A few drops of this oil in a hot shower can help to clear sinuses, relieve congestion, and open up the airways. It can also be added to bathwater to create a relaxing and refreshing soak.

Eucalyptus oil is also commonly used in massage therapy. Its cooling and soothing properties make it an ideal oil for reducing muscle tension and soreness. When mixed with a carrier oil such as almond or jojoba oil, eucalyptus oil can be applied directly to the skin for a relaxing and invigorating massage.

Fragrance Oils for Home Décor: Enhancing Your Living Space with Scent

In addition to its therapeutic benefits, eucalyptus oil is also a popular choice for home décor. Its fresh, clean scent makes it a great oil for use in candles, room sprays, and diffusers. It can be blended with other oils such as lavender or peppermint to create a unique and refreshing fragrance for any room in the house.

When shopping for eucalyptus oil, it is important to choose a high-quality, pure essential oil. Look for oils that have been steam distilled from the leaves of the eucalyptus tree, and avoid oils that have been extracted using harsh chemicals or solvents.

Overall, eucalyptus is a versatile and refreshing fragrance oil that can enhance the ambiance of any living space. Whether for aromatherapy or home décor, this essential oil is a must-have for any fragrance collection.

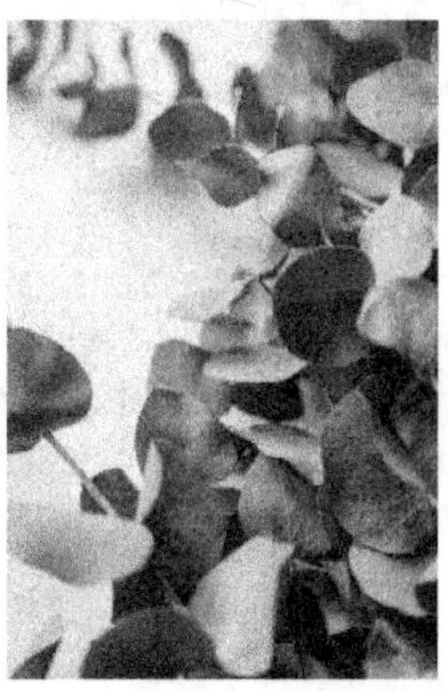

Rose

Rose fragrance oil is one of the most popular scents in aromatherapy essential and fragrance oils. It is often referred to as the queen of flowers, and its fragrance is associated with love, beauty, and femininity.

Rose fragrance oil is extracted from the petals of the rose flower, and it has a sweet, floral scent that is both calming and uplifting. The oil is known for its therapeutic properties, and it is often used in aromatherapy to help reduce anxiety, promote relaxation, and enhance mood.

In home décor, rose fragrance oil is a popular choice for creating a romantic and inviting atmosphere. It can be used in a variety of ways, including as a room spray, in candles, or in diffusers. Rose fragrance oil can also be added to bath products, such as soaps and bath salts, to create a luxurious spa-like experience at home.

When selecting a rose fragrance oil, it is important to choose high-quality oils that are free of synthetic fragrances and chemicals. Look for oils that are made from natural ingredients and are certified organic, if possible.

Fragrance Oils for Home Décor: Enhancing Your Living Space with Scent

To use rose fragrance oil in your home, simply add a few drops to a diffuser or mix with water in a spray bottle to create a room spray. You can also add a few drops of the oil to a warm bath to create a relaxing and soothing experience.

Overall, rose fragrance oil is a versatile and popular scent that can enhance any living space with its beautiful aroma and therapeutic properties. Whether you are looking to create a romantic atmosphere in your bedroom or promote relaxation in your living room, rose fragrance oil is a great choice for enhancing your home décor with scent.

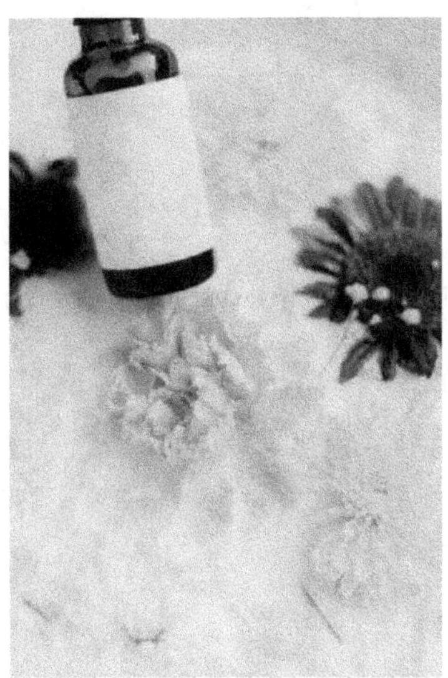

Vanilla

Vanilla is a popular fragrance oil used in aromatherapy, home décor, and personal care products. Its sweet and comforting scent is known for its ability to reduce stress and anxiety, promote relaxation, and improve mood.

Vanilla fragrance oil is extracted from the vanilla bean, a type of orchid that grows in tropical climates. The process of extracting vanilla fragrance oil involves drying and curing the vanilla beans, then soaking them in a solvent to extract the aromatic compounds. The resulting oil can be used in a variety of ways, including in diffusers, candles, bath and body products, and even in cooking.

One of the most popular uses for vanilla fragrance oil is in diffusers. Adding a few drops of vanilla oil to a diffuser can create a warm and inviting atmosphere in your home. Vanilla oil is also often used in candles, either on its own or combined with other fragrances like cinnamon or lavender. The scent of vanilla can help to create a cozy and comforting ambiance, perfect for relaxing after a long day.

Fragrance Oils for Home Décor: Enhancing Your Living Space with Scent

In addition to its use in home décor, vanilla fragrance oil is also commonly used in personal care products like lotions, soaps, and body sprays. The scent of vanilla is believed to have aphrodisiac properties, making it a popular choice for romantic gifts like massage oils and perfumes.

When shopping for vanilla fragrance oil, it's important to choose a high-quality product that is pure and free of synthetic fragrances. Look for products that are labeled as "100% pure vanilla oil" and avoid those that contain additives or fillers.

Overall, vanilla fragrance oil is a versatile and comforting scent that can enhance your living space and promote relaxation and well-being. Whether you're using it in a diffuser, candle, or personal care product, the sweet and soothing aroma of vanilla is sure to bring a sense of warmth and comfort to your home.

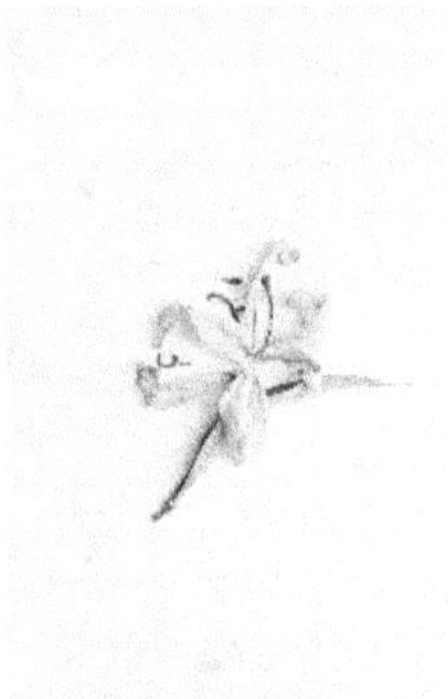

Cinnamon

Cinnamon has been used for centuries in traditional medicine to treat a variety of ailments. It is believed to have anti-inflammatory and antioxidant properties, making it a popular choice for aromatherapy. When inhaled, the warm and spicy aroma of cinnamon can help relieve stress and anxiety, improve mood, and promote relaxation.

Cinnamon is a beloved spice with a warm, comforting aroma that is often associated with the holiday season. However, cinnamon is more than just a kitchen staple. It is a powerful ingredient in aromatherapy and fragrance oils that can enhance the ambiance of any living space. In this subchapter, we will explore the many benefits of cinnamon and how it can be used in the home.

In addition to its therapeutic benefits, cinnamon is a versatile fragrance oil that can be used in a variety of home décor applications. It can be used to create a warm and inviting atmosphere in a living room or bedroom, or to add a spicy kick to a kitchen or dining room.

One of the most popular ways to use cinnamon in fragrance oils is in candles. Cinnamon candles are a favorite during the fall and winter months, but they can be enjoyed year-round.

Fragrance Oils for Home Décor: Enhancing Your Living Space with Scent

They can be used to create a cozy ambiance in a living space or to add a touch of elegance to a special occasion.

Cinnamon can also be used in diffusers and room sprays. Diffusers are a great way to enjoy the therapeutic benefits of cinnamon throughout the day, while room sprays can be used to freshen up a space and add a burst of fragrance.

When using cinnamon fragrance oils, it is important to choose high-quality oils that are free of synthetic additives and chemicals. Look for oils that are made from pure cinnamon essential oil or natural cinnamon extracts.

Cinnamon is a powerful fragrance oil that can enhance the ambiance of any living space. Whether you prefer candles, diffusers, or room sprays, cinnamon is a versatile ingredient that can be enjoyed year-round. So why not add a touch of warm and spicy goodness to your home décor today?

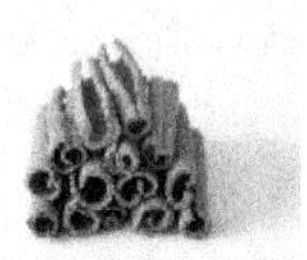

Lemon

Lemon is one of the most popular and widely used fragrance oils in home décor. It has a fresh, uplifting scent that can brighten up any living space and create a sense of cleanliness and freshness. The scent of lemon is known to have a positive effect on mood and can help to reduce stress and anxiety.

In aromatherapy, lemon is often used to promote feelings of clarity and focus. It is believed to have a purifying effect on the mind, helping to clear away mental fog and improve concentration. This makes it an ideal fragrance oil to use in your office or study area.

Lemon fragrance oil is also a great choice for the kitchen. Its fresh, clean scent can help to eliminate unwanted odors and create a pleasant atmosphere while cooking and entertaining guests. Simply add a few drops of lemon oil to a diffuser or oil burner to create a welcoming and refreshing environment.

When it comes to home cleaning, lemon oil is a powerful natural cleaner that can be used to clean and sanitize surfaces around the house. Its antiseptic properties make it an ideal ingredient in natural cleaning products, and it can also be added to laundry detergent to help remove stubborn stains and odors.

Fragrance Oils for Home Décor: Enhancing Your Living Space with Scent

In addition to its many practical uses, lemon fragrance oil is also a popular choice for creating scented candles, soaps, and bath products. Its fresh, citrusy scent is a favorite among both men and women, making it a versatile fragrance oil that can be used in a variety of home décor and personal care products.

Whether you are looking to enhance your living space with a fresh, uplifting scent or simply enjoy the many benefits of lemon fragrance oil, there are plenty of ways to incorporate this versatile scent into your home décor and daily routine.

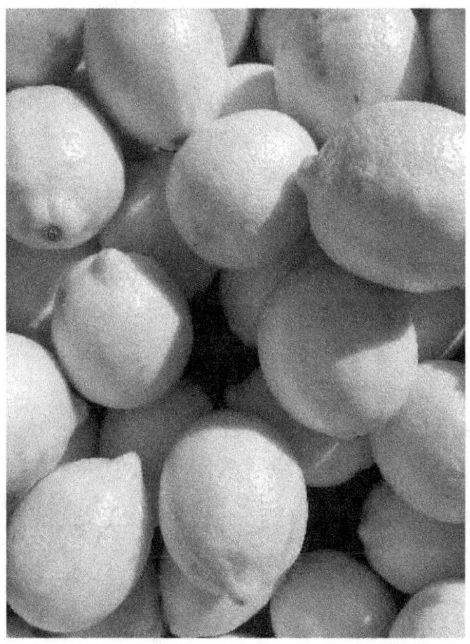

Fragrance Oils for Home Décor: Enhancing Your Living Space with Scent

Orange

Orange is one of the most popular and versatile fragrances used in aromatherapy essential and fragrance oils. Its warm and invigorating scent can help uplift your mood, reduce stress and anxiety, and improve your overall well-being.

Orange essential oil is extracted from the peel of the orange fruit and contains powerful antioxidants and anti-inflammatory properties. It is also rich in vitamins and minerals that can help improve your skin's texture and appearance.

In home décor, orange fragrance oils can add a burst of freshness and energy to any room. They are perfect for creating a warm and welcoming atmosphere in your living space. You can use them in diffusers, candles, or potpourri to create a refreshing and invigorating ambiance.

One of the best ways to use orange fragrance oils is to mix them with other essential oils. Lavender, peppermint, and eucalyptus oils can complement the citrusy scent of orange and create a more complex and appealing fragrance. You can experiment with different combinations to find the perfect blend that suits your taste and mood.

Fragrance Oils for Home Décor: Enhancing Your Living Space with Scent

Orange fragrance oils are also ideal for creating homemade cleaning products. They have natural antibacterial and antifungal properties that can help keep your home clean and fresh-smelling. You can add a few drops of orange oil to your cleaning solution or use it as a room spray to keep your home smelling clean and invigorating.

Orange fragrance oils are a must-have in any aromatherapy essential and fragrance oil collection. They offer a wide range of benefits for your physical and mental health, and they can enhance your home décor with their warm and energizing scent. Whether you're looking to improve your mood, reduce stress, or freshen up your living space, orange fragrance oils are a versatile and effective solution.

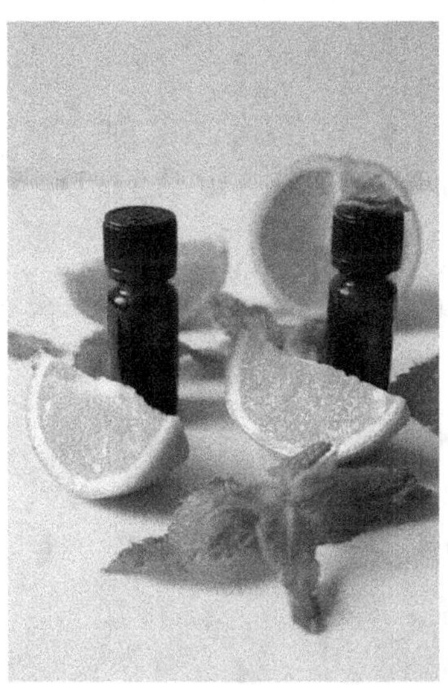

Fragrance Oils for Home Décor: Enhancing Your Living Space with Scent

Sandalwood

Sandalwood is one of the most popular and widely used scents in the world of aromatherapy essential and fragrance oils. It has a warm, woody, and exotic aroma that is both calming and uplifting. The scent of sandalwood is derived from the wood of the Santalum tree, which is native to India, Indonesia, and Australia.

Sandalwood has been used for centuries in traditional Ayurvedic medicine for its therapeutic properties. It is known to have a calming effect on the mind and body and is often used in meditation to promote relaxation and inner peace. Sandalwood is also believed to have aphrodisiac properties and is often used in perfumes and colognes.

In addition to its therapeutic properties, sandalwood is also a popular choice for home decor. It can be used in a variety of ways to enhance the ambiance of your living space. One popular way to use sandalwood is to add a few drops of sandalwood essential oil to a diffuser or oil burner. This will help to fill your home with the warm and inviting scent of sandalwood.

Another way to use sandalwood in home decor is to add it to your cleaning products. You can add a few drops of sandalwood essential oil to your laundry detergent, fabric softener, or cleaning spray to give your home a fresh and inviting scent.

Fragrance Oils for Home Décor: Enhancing Your Living Space with Scent

Sandalwood is also a popular choice for candles and incense. The warm and inviting scent of sandalwood can help to create a relaxing and peaceful atmosphere in your home. You can find a variety of sandalwood scented candles and incense at your local home decor store or online.

InSandalwood is a versatile and popular scent that can be used in a variety of ways to enhance your home decor. Whether you are looking for a calming scent for your meditation practice or a warm and inviting scent for your living space, sandalwood is a great choice. So why not add a touch of sandalwood to your home decor today?

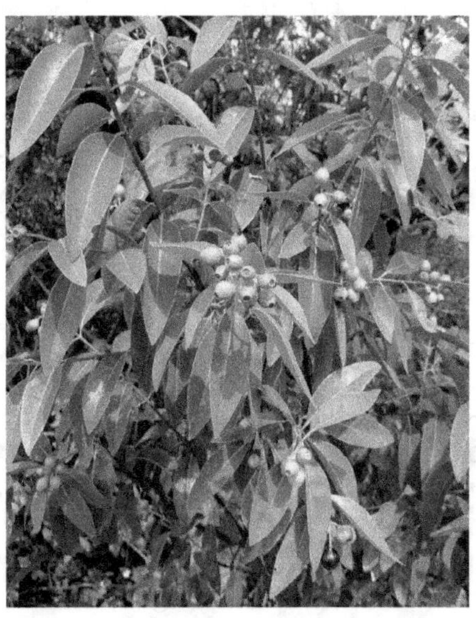

Tips and Tricks for Using Fragrance Oils in Home Décor

How to mix and match fragrance oils

When it comes to enhancing your living space with fragrance oils, there are countless options to choose from. However, mixing and matching these oils can be a slightly more complex process. Here are a few tips to help you mix and match fragrance oils like a pro.

1. Start with a Base Note

Every fragrance oil has a base note, middle note, and top note. The base note is the scent that lingers the longest and provides the foundation for your fragrance blend. Start by selecting a base note that you love and build your fragrance blend from there.

2. Add a Middle Note

The middle note is the scent that provides depth and body to your fragrance blend. It usually lasts for a few hours and helps to balance out the base note. Common middle notes include lavender, cinnamon, and rosemary.

Fragrance Oils for Home Décor: Enhancing Your Living Space with Scent

3. Finish with a Top Note

The top note is the scent that you smell first and it usually lasts for just a few minutes. It provides a burst of freshness to your fragrance blend and can be used to add a little extra something to your fragrance. Common top notes include lemon, bergamot, and peppermint.

4. Experiment with Ratios

The ratio of base, middle, and top notes in your fragrance blend is crucial to achieving the perfect scent. Start with a 2:1:1 ratio of base note to middle note to top note and adjust as needed until you find the perfect balance.

5. Don't Be Afraid to Mix and Match

Mixing and matching fragrance oils can be a lot of fun, so don't be afraid to experiment. Try blending different scents together until you find the perfect combination for your home décor.

In conclusion, mixing and matching fragrance oils can be a great way to create a unique and inviting scent for your home. Keep these tips in mind and don't be afraid to get creative with your fragrance blends. Happy blending!

How to store fragrance oils

Fragrance oils are an essential part of home décor, with their ability to evoke emotions and create a comfortable atmosphere in any living space. However, proper storage of these oils is crucial to ensure their longevity and effectiveness. In this subchapter, we will discuss some practical tips on how to store fragrance oils to maintain their quality and aroma.

Firstly, it is vital to store fragrance oils in a cool, dry, and dark place. Direct sunlight and high temperatures can cause the oils to deteriorate quickly, resulting in a loss of scent and potency. A dark cabinet or drawer away from any heat sources is an ideal storage solution.

Secondly, it is essential to keep fragrance oils in airtight glass bottles or vials. Exposure to air can cause the oils to oxidize and lose their fragrance over time. Glass bottles are preferable as they do not react with the oils as plastic containers can. Also, ensure that the lids of the bottles are tightly sealed to prevent any air from seeping in.

Amber or dark coloured PET bottles are also used to store fragrance oils.

Fragrance Oils for Home Décor: Enhancing Your Living Space with Scent

Thirdly, it is essential to label your fragrance oils clearly. It can be challenging to identify specific oils once they are stored away, especially if you have a collection of many different scents. Labeling the bottles with the name of the oil and the date of purchase can help you keep track of their freshness and avoid using expired oils.

Lastly, keep your fragrance oils away from children and pets. They can be hazardous if ingested or applied directly to the skin. Store them in a high and secure location, out of reach of curious little hands and paws.

Proper storage of fragrance oils is crucial to preserve their scent and potency. Ensure that they are stored in a cool, dry, and dark place in airtight glass bottles, labeled correctly, and kept away from children and pets. By following these simple steps, you can enjoy the full benefits of your fragrance oils for a long time.

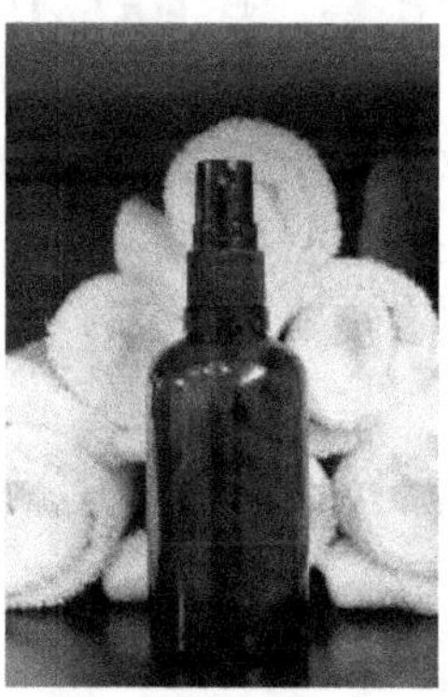

How to adjust the strength of fragrance oils

Fragrance oils are an essential part of aromatherapy, and they are used in a variety of ways to enhance the ambiance of living spaces, promote relaxation, and improve mood. The strength of fragrance oils is an important consideration when using them, as it determines the intensity of the scent and the effectiveness of the aromatherapy.

To adjust the strength of fragrance oils, there are several factors to consider, such as the type of oil, the concentration, and the method of application. Here are some tips to help you adjust the strength of your fragrance oils and achieve the desired results:

1. Choose the Right Concentration

Fragrance oils come in different concentrations, ranging from 1% to 20%, depending on the type and quality of the oil. The higher the concentration, the stronger the scent, and the more effective the aromatherapy. However, high concentrations of fragrance oils can also be overwhelming and cause headaches or allergic reactions. Therefore, it's important to choose the right concentration based on your preferences and sensitivity.

2. Dilute the Oil

Fragrance Oils for Home Décor: Enhancing Your Living Space with Scent

If the fragrance oil is too strong, you can dilute it with a carrier oil, such as almond, coconut, or jojoba oil. This will reduce the concentration and intensity of the scent while preserving its therapeutic properties. The ratio of fragrance oil to carrier oil depends on the desired strength of the scent, but a good starting point is 1-2 drops of fragrance oil per teaspoon of carrier oil.

3. Adjust the Application Method

The method of application also affects the strength of fragrance oils. For example, diffusing the oil in a large room will require more drops than applying it directly to the skin. If the scent is too strong, you can reduce the number of drops or switch to a milder application method, such as using a room spray or a reed diffuser.

4. Experiment with Blends

Blending different fragrance oils can also help you adjust the strength and achieve a unique scent profile. For example, adding a few drops of lavender oil to a citrus blend can balance the intensity and promote relaxation. Experiment with different blends and ratios until you find the perfect balance for your needs.

Fragrance Oils for Home Décor: Enhancing Your Living Space with Scent

In conclusion, adjusting the strength of fragrance oils is a simple but important step in using them effectively for aromatherapy and home decor. By considering the concentration, dilution, application method, and blending options, you can customize the scent to your preferences and enjoy the benefits of aromatherapy in your living space.

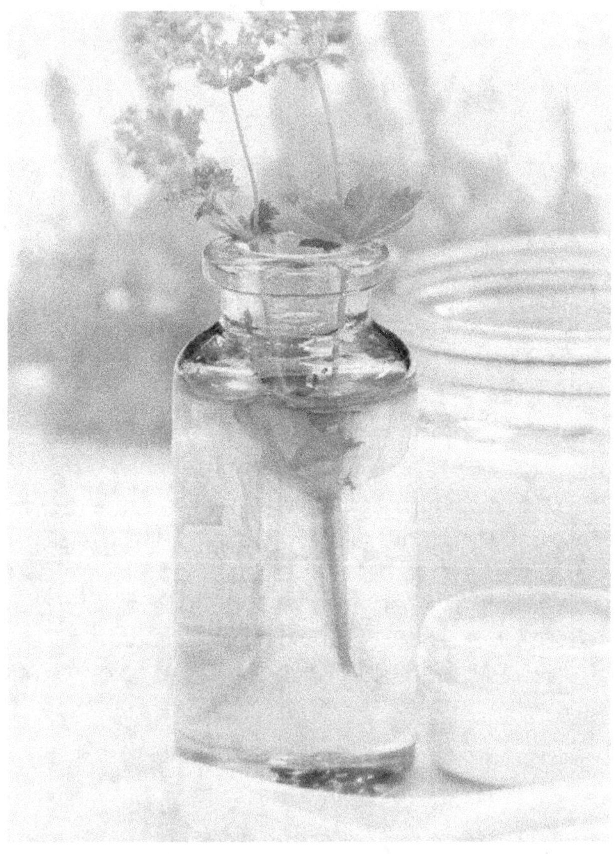

Fragrance Oils for Home Décor: Enhancing Your Living Space with Scent

How to create a signature scent for your home

Creating a signature scent for your home is a fun and creative way to add a personal touch to your living space. A signature scent can create a welcoming and inviting atmosphere that reflects your personality and style. Here are some tips on how to create a signature scent for your home using fragrance oils.

1. Determine the mood you want to create

Before you start mixing fragrance oils, think about the mood you want to create in your home. Do you want a relaxing and calming atmosphere, or do you prefer a vibrant and energizing one? The mood you want to create will help you choose the right fragrance oils for your signature scent.

2. Choose your fragrance oils

Once you have determined the mood you want to create, it's time to choose your fragrance oils. Aromatherapy essential oils are a great option if you want to create a calming and relaxing atmosphere. Lavender, chamomile, and bergamot are great choices for this. If you want a more energizing atmosphere, citrus oils like lemon, grapefruit, and orange are perfect.

Fragrance Oils for Home Décor: Enhancing Your Living Space with Scent

3. Mix and match

Mixing and matching different fragrance oils is the key to creating a signature scent that is unique and personal. Start by mixing a few drops of your chosen oils in a spray bottle filled with water. Spray the mixture in different areas of your home and see how it smells. Once you have found the right combination, you can mix a larger batch of your signature scent.

4. Experiment with different scents

Don't be afraid to experiment with different scents until you find the perfect combination for your signature scent. You can also try adding other scents like vanilla or cinnamon to create a warm and cozy atmosphere.

Creating a signature scent for your home is a simple and affordable way to enhance your living space with scent. With these tips, you can create a signature scent that reflects your personality and style.

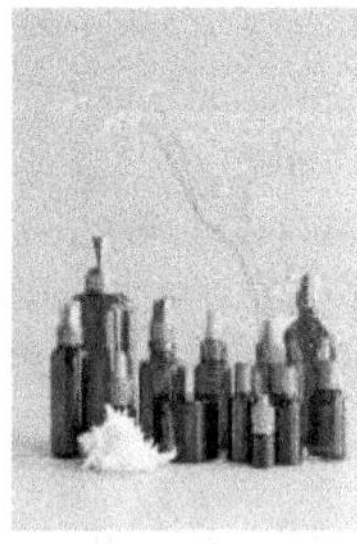

Risks and Precautions of Using Fragrance Oils

Possible allergic reactions to fragrance oils

Possible allergic reactions to fragrance oils

Fragrance oils are a great way to add a pleasant fragrance to your home, office, or any other living space. However, some people may experience allergic reactions to certain types of fragrance oils. This is why it is important to be aware of the possible allergic reactions that can occur when using fragrance oils.

Skin irritation

One of the most common allergic reactions to fragrance oils is skin irritation. This can manifest as itching, redness, or even a rash. If you notice any of these symptoms after using a fragrance oil, it is best to stop using it immediately.

Respiratory problems

Fragrance Oils for Home Décor: Enhancing Your Living Space with Scent

Another common allergic reaction to fragrance oils is respiratory problems. This can include coughing, wheezing, and difficulty breathing. If you experience any of these symptoms, it is important to seek medical attention immediately.

Headaches

Some people may also experience headaches after using certain types of fragrance oils. This is because certain fragrances can trigger migraines or other types of headaches.

Allergic reactions can vary from person to person, and some people may be more sensitive to certain types of fragrance oils than others. It is always best to test a small amount of the fragrance oil on your skin before using it extensively. If you notice any adverse reactions, it is best to stop using the fragrance oil immediately.

While fragrance oils can be a great way to enhance your living space with scent, it is important to be aware of the possible allergic reactions that can occur. By being aware of these potential reactions, you can help ensure that you are using fragrance oils safely and responsibly.

How to test for allergies

As a retail end user of aromatherapy essential and fragrance oils, it is essential to understand how to test for allergies before using any new product. Allergies can cause a range of symptoms, from skin irritation to respiratory issues, so it is crucial to take the necessary precautions to keep yourself safe.

The first step in testing for allergies is to perform a patch test. To do this, simply apply a small amount of the oil to an inconspicuous area of skin, such as the inside of your elbow or wrist. Wait for at least 24 hours to see if any redness, itching, or swelling occurs. If there is no reaction, it is likely safe to use the oil as intended.

If you do experience a reaction, it is best to avoid using the product altogether. However, if you are determined to use the oil, consider diluting it with a carrier oil to reduce its potency. This can help minimize the risk of an allergic reaction.

Another option is to perform a nasal inhalation test. This involves placing a drop of the oil on a tissue or cotton ball and holding it close to your nose. Inhale deeply and observe any symptoms, such as sneezing, coughing, or congestion. If you experience any adverse effects, it is best to avoid using the oil.

Fragrance Oils for Home Décor: Enhancing Your Living Space with Scent

It is also essential to be aware of any preexisting allergies or sensitivities you may have. If you are allergic to a particular plant or substance, it is possible that you may also be allergic to the essential oil derived from that source. Always read the label and research the ingredients before using any new product.

Testing for allergies is a crucial step in using aromatherapy essential and fragrance oils safely. Always perform a patch test or nasal inhalation test before using a new product, and be aware of any preexisting allergies or sensitivities. By taking these precautions, you can enjoy the benefits of aromatherapy without putting your health at risk.

The importance of using fragrance oils properly

The importance of using fragrance oils properly cannot be overstated. Fragrance oils are concentrated scents that are used to enhance the ambiance of living spaces, but they must be used in the right way to get the desired effect. Here are some tips on how to use fragrance oils properly.

First and foremost, it is important to use high-quality fragrance oils. The fragrance oil market is flooded with cheap, synthetic oils that can be harmful to your health and the environment. Look for fragrance oils that are made from natural ingredients and are free from harmful chemicals.

When using fragrance oils, it is important to use them sparingly. Fragrance oils are highly concentrated, and a little goes a long way. Start with just a few drops and gradually increase the amount until you achieve the desired scent.

Another important factor to consider when using fragrance oils is the method of application. There are several ways to use fragrance oils, including diffusers, candles, and sprays. Each method has its own benefits and drawbacks, so it is important to choose the right method for your needs.

Fragrance Oils for Home Décor: Enhancing Your Living Space with Scent

Diffusers are a popular method of using fragrance oils because they release a consistent scent into the air. They come in different types, such as electric diffusers, reed diffusers, and ultrasonic diffusers. Candles are also a popular method of using fragrance oils, but they require more attention and can be a fire hazard. Sprays are a quick and easy way to freshen up a room, but they do not last as long as other methods.

Using fragrance oils properly is essential for creating a welcoming and inviting living space. By choosing high-quality oils, using them sparingly, and choosing the right method of application, you can enjoy the benefits of fragrance oils without any negative side effects.

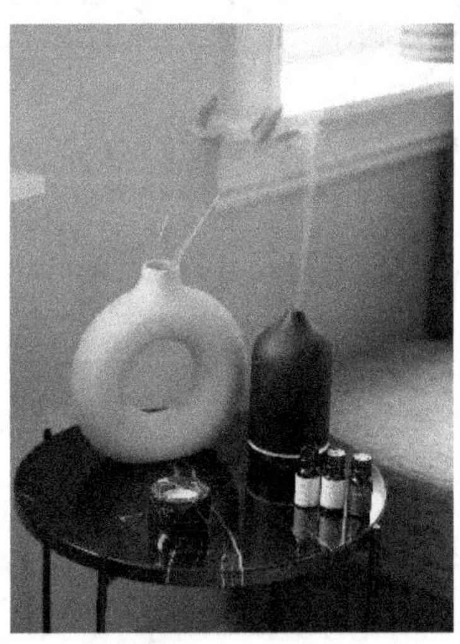

How to safely store fragrance oils

Fragrance oils are a popular choice for many people who want to enhance the scent of their living space. Whether you are using them for aromatherapy, relaxation, or simply to create a pleasant atmosphere, it is important to know how to store these oils safely.

Firstly, it is important to keep fragrance oils in a cool, dark place. Exposure to light and heat can cause the oils to break down, which can lead to a loss of fragrance or even spoilage. It is best to store your oils in a cabinet or drawer, away from direct sunlight and heat sources.

It is also important to keep fragrance oils away from children and pets. While these oils are safe for use in your home, they can be harmful if ingested or applied directly to the skin. To prevent accidents, be sure to store your oils in a secure, out-of-reach location.

When storing fragrance oils, it is also important to keep them in their original containers. This is because many oils are sensitive to air, and exposure to oxygen can cause them to lose their potency.

If you do need to transfer your oils to a different container, be sure to use a dark glass bottle with a tight-fitting lid.

Fragrance Oils for Home Décor: Enhancing Your Living Space with Scent

Finally, it is important to label your fragrance oils properly. This will help you to keep track of which oils you have and when they were purchased, which can be helpful for tracking shelf life. It can also prevent confusion if you have multiple oils with similar scents.

Proper storage of fragrance oils is essential to maintaining their potency and ensuring their safety. Keep them in a cool, dark place, away from children and pets, in their original containers, and label them properly. By following these simple tips, you can enjoy the benefits of fragrance oils for years to come.

Recap of the benefits and uses of fragrance oils in home décor

Fragrance oils have been used for centuries to add a touch of luxury and comfort to living spaces. In recent times, their popularity has increased as people have become more aware of the benefits of aromatherapy and the positive impact of fragrances on our emotional well-being. In this subchapter, we will recap the benefits and uses of fragrance oils in home décor.

Firstly, fragrance oils are an excellent way to create a welcoming and inviting atmosphere in your home. A carefully chosen fragrance can evoke memories, create a calming environment, or even stimulate the senses. Some common fragrances used in home décor include lavender for relaxation, peppermint for energy, and citrus for a refreshing scent.

Another use of fragrance oils is to mask unpleasant odors in your home. By using a diffuser or reed diffuser, you can fill your living space with a pleasant scent that will help to neutralize any unwanted smells. This is particularly useful in areas such as the kitchen, bathroom, or pet areas.

Fragrance Oils for Home Décor: Enhancing Your Living Space with Scent

Fragrance oils can also be used to enhance your home décor. A beautifully designed diffuser or candle can be a statement piece in any room, while also adding a touch of elegance and sophistication. Additionally, fragrance oils can be used in potpourri, sachets, or even in homemade cleaning products to add a touch of fragrance to your daily routine.

One of the most significant benefits of fragrance oils is their positive impact on our emotional well-being. Aromatherapy essential and fragrance oils have been shown to reduce stress, anxiety, and even depression. By using these oils in your home décor, you can create a calming and relaxing environment that promotes a sense of well-being and tranquility.

Fragrance oils are an excellent way to enhance your living space with scent. Whether you are looking to create a welcoming atmosphere, mask unpleasant odors, or promote emotional well-being, fragrance oils offer a wide range of benefits and uses. With so many fragrances and diffuser options available, you are sure to find the perfect combination to suit your personal style and needs.

Tips for getting started with using fragrance oils

Tips for Getting Started with Using Fragrance Oils

Fragrance oils are an essential part of any aromatherapy or home décor routine. They can be used to create a calming and relaxing atmosphere in your living space, or to freshen up your home with a delightful scent. If you are new to using fragrance oils, here are some tips to help you get started.

1. Choose the right fragrance oil for your needs:

When selecting a fragrance oil, consider the purpose for which you want to use it. Are you looking for a relaxing scent to use in your bedroom, or a refreshing scent for your kitchen? Different oils have different properties and can be used for a variety of purposes. Some are uplifting and energizing, while others are calming and soothing. Take the time to research and choose the right fragrance oil for your needs.

2. Use the right tools:

Fragrance Oils for Home Décor: Enhancing Your Living Space with Scent

To get the best results from your fragrance oils, it is important to use the right tools.

One of the most popular methods of using fragrance oils is through a diffuser, so use diffuser tools to create your preferred scent for your home. There are many types of diffusers available, from electric diffusers to reed diffusers. Choose the one that best suits your needs and the size of your room.

3. Don't overdo it:

While fragrance oils can create a beautiful scent in your home, it is important not to overdo it. Too much fragrance can be overwhelming and even trigger headaches or other reactions. Start with a small amount of oil and gradually increase the amount until you find the perfect balance.

4. Experiment with blending:

One of the great things about fragrance oils is that they can be blended to create your own unique scent. Experiment with different blends to find the perfect combination for your home. Start by blending two or three oils together and adjust the amounts until you find the perfect balance.

Fragrance Oils for Home Décor: Enhancing Your Living Space with Scent

5. Store your oils properly:

Fragrance oils should be stored properly to maintain their potency and fragrance. Store them in a cool, dark place away from direct sunlight and heat. This will help to preserve the oils and ensure that they last for as long as possible.

Using fragrance oils can be a wonderful way to enhance your living space with scent. By following these tips, you can get started with using fragrance oils and create a beautiful and inviting atmosphere in your home.

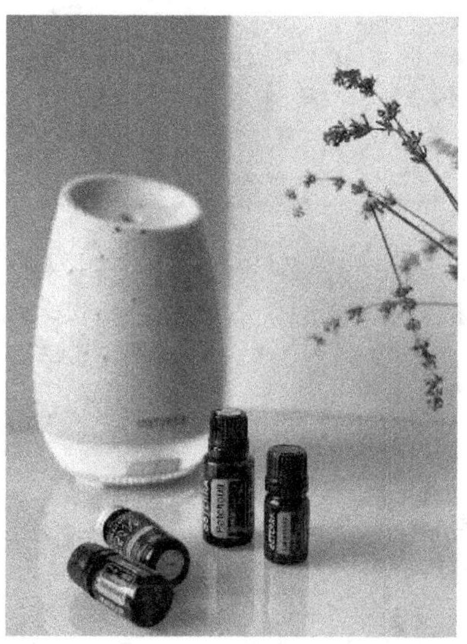

Resources for purchasing fragrance oils and accessories

When it comes to enhancing your living space with fragrance oils, one of the most important things you need to know is where to purchase the right oils and accessories. Luckily, there are plenty of resources available to help you find the best products for your needs.

One of the best places to start your search is online. There are countless online retailers that specialize in fragrance oils and accessories, catering to a wide range of needs and preferences. Some of the most popular online retailers include Ebay, Amazon, Etsy, and FragranceNet. These retailers offer a variety of different types of fragrance oils, including essential oils, fragrance oils, and blends.

They also offer a range of accessories, such as diffusers, candles, and room sprays, which can help you get the most out of your fragrance oils.

Another great resource for purchasing fragrance oils and accessories is your local health food store. Many health food stores carry a variety of essential oils and fragrance oils, as well as diffusers and other accessories. This can be a great option if you prefer to shop in person and want to support local businesses.

Fragrance Oils for Home Décor: Enhancing Your Living Space with Scent

If you're looking for high-quality, organic fragrance oils, you may want to consider visiting a specialty store. These stores typically offer a smaller selection of products but focus on quality over quantity. They may also offer personalized consultations to help you find the right fragrance oils for your needs.

Finally, if you're interested in creating your own fragrance blends, you may want to consider purchasing individual essential oils and blending them yourself. Many online retailers and specialty stores offer a wide range of essential oils, which can be used alone or combined to create unique fragrance blends.

Overall, there are plenty of resources available to help you find the right fragrance oils and accessories for your needs. Whether you prefer to shop online or in person, there are plenty of options to choose from, so don't be afraid to explore and find the products that work best for you.

Appendix

Glossary of terms

As you dive deeper into the world of fragrance oils for home décor, you may come across terms that are unfamiliar to you. To help you better understand the terminology used in the industry, we have compiled a glossary of terms for your reference.

Aromatherapy - The practice of using essential oils from plants to promote physical and emotional well-being.

Carrier Oil - A neutral oil used to dilute essential oils before they are applied to the skin.

Diffuser - A device that disperses fragrance into the air, typically using heat, evaporation, or ultrasonic technology.

Essential Oil - A concentrated liquid extracted from plants that contains the aroma and therapeutic properties of the plant.

Fragrance Oils for Home Décor: Enhancing Your Living Space with Scent

Fragrance Oil - A synthetic or natural oil that is used to add scent to products such as candles, soaps, and lotions.

Inhalation - The process of breathing in fragrance molecules through the nose or mouth, which can have a therapeutic effect on the body and mind.

Nebulizer - A type of diffuser that uses high-pressure air to break up essential oils into small particles for inhalation.

Perfume Oil - A concentrated fragrance oil that is used to create perfumes and colognes.

Scent Throw - The distance that a fragrance can be detected from its source.

Top Note - The initial scent that is detected when a fragrance is first applied, typically lasting for only a few minutes.

Middle Note - The scent that emerges after the top note dissipates, also known as the heart note.

Base Note - The scent that remains after the top and middle notes have evaporated, typically lasting for several hours.

Fragrance Oils for Home Décor: Enhancing Your Living Space with Scent

With this glossary of terms, you will be better equipped to understand the language of the fragrance oil industry.

Whether you are looking to enhance your living space with scent or explore the therapeutic benefits of aromatherapy essential oils, these terms will help you navigate the world of fragrance with confidence.

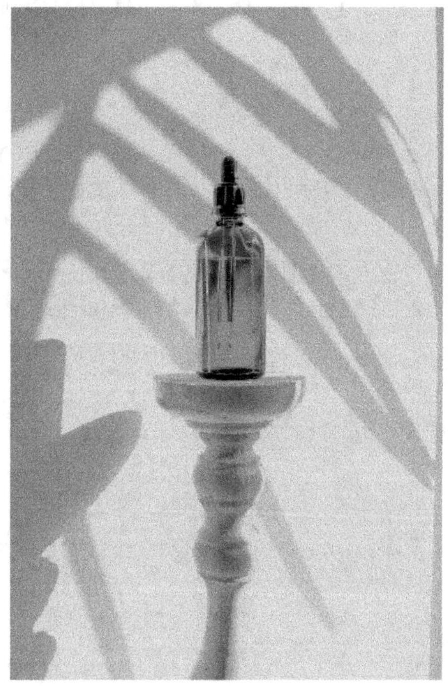

Fragrance Oils for Home Décor: Enhancing Your Living Space with Scent

List of suppliers of fragrance oils and accessories

When it comes to creating a welcoming and inviting atmosphere in your home, fragrance oils are a must-have. They not only infuse your living space with beautiful scents but also have therapeutic properties that can help promote relaxation and calmness. However, with so many suppliers offering different types of fragrance oils and accessories, it can be challenging to know where to start. Here is a list of some of the best suppliers for fragrance oils and accessories that will help you create a serene living space.

1. EOOC Essential Oils

EOOC Oils is a family run business who are popular suppliers of essential oils and fragrance oils, and they are known for their high-quality products. They offer a wide range of fragrance oils, including single oils, blends, and seasonal scents. Their oils are 100% pure and free from any synthetic additives, making them perfect for aromatherapy use.

2. Natures Garden

Fragrance Oils for Home Décor: Enhancing Your Living Space with Scent

Natures Garden is another reputable supplier of fragrance oils and accessories. They offer over 800 different fragrance oils, including unique scents like Bubble Gum and Blueberry Cheesecake. They also offer a range of accessories like diffusers, bottles, and wicks that will help you get the most out of your fragrance oils.

3. CandleScience

If you are looking for fragrance oils specifically for candle making, CandleScience is the perfect supplier. They offer a range of candle fragrances that are perfect for creating beautiful scented candles. They also offer a range of candle-making supplies like waxes, wicks, and containers, making it easy to create your own candles at home.

4. Essican Purelife

Essican Purelife is a one-stop-factory for all your fragrance oil and accessory needs. They offer a wide range of fragrance oils, including natural and organic options. They also offer a range of accessories like diffusers, bottles, and packaging supplies that will help you create beautiful scented products.

5. White Rose Essential Oils

Fragrance Oils for Home Décor: Enhancing Your Living Space with Scent

White Rose Essential Oils is a family-owned business that has been supplying fragrance oils and accessories for over 30 years. They offer a range of fragrance oils, including unique scents like Rainforest and Sandalwood Vanilla. They also offer a range of accessories like diffusers, burners, and incense sticks that will help you create a relaxing and calming atmosphere in your home.

In conclusion, when it comes to purchasing fragrance oils and accessories, it's essential to choose a reputable supplier that offers high-quality products. The suppliers listed above are some of the best in the industry and will help you create a beautiful and inviting living space with their fragrance oils and accessories.

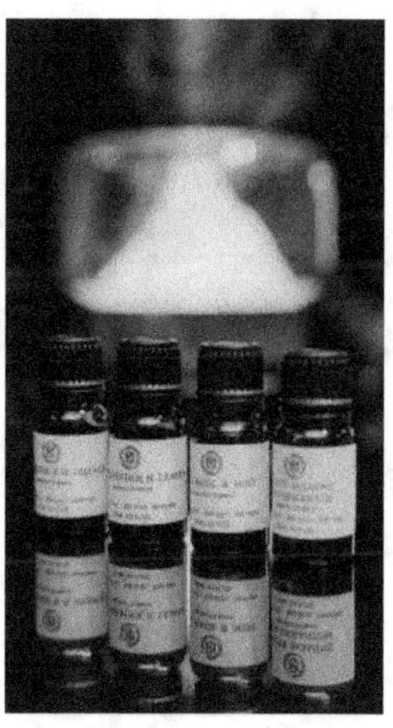

Frequently asked questions about fragrance oils

Frequently asked questions about fragrance oils

Fragrance oils are a popular choice for those looking to enhance the ambiance of their living space with a pleasant scent. As a retail end user, you may have some questions about fragrance oils, including their uses, benefits, and safety. In this section, we'll answer some of the most frequently asked questions about fragrance oils.

1. What are fragrance oils, and how are they different from essential oils?

Fragrance oils are synthetic or natural blends of aromatic compounds that are designed to mimic the scent of natural substances. They are typically used for their scent, rather than for their therapeutic properties. Essential oils, on the other hand, are concentrated extracts from plants that are used for their therapeutic benefits, as well as their scent.

2. How can fragrance oils be used?

Fragrance Oils for Home Décor: Enhancing Your Living Space with Scent

Fragrance oils can be used in a variety of ways, including in fragrance diffusers, candles, soaps, lotions, and other personal care products. They can also be added to cleaning products, laundry detergents, and other household items to provide a pleasant scent.

3. What are the benefits of fragrance oils?

Fragrance oils can provide a variety of benefits, including improving mood, reducing stress, and promoting relaxation. They can also help to eliminate unpleasant odors and create a welcoming atmosphere in your home.

4. Are fragrance oils safe to use?

When used as directed, fragrance oils are generally considered safe. However, it's important to follow the instructions on the product label and avoid direct skin contact with undiluted oils. Some fragrance oils may also contain allergens or irritants, so it's a good idea to test a small amount before using them extensively.

5. How should fragrance oils be stored?

Fragrance oils should be stored in a cool, dark place away from heat and light. They should also be kept out of reach of children and pets.

Fragrance Oils for Home Décor: Enhancing Your Living Space with Scent

In conclusion, fragrance oils can be a great choice for enhancing the ambiance of your living space with a pleasant scent. By following the instructions on the product label and using them safely, you can enjoy their benefits without any negative side effects.

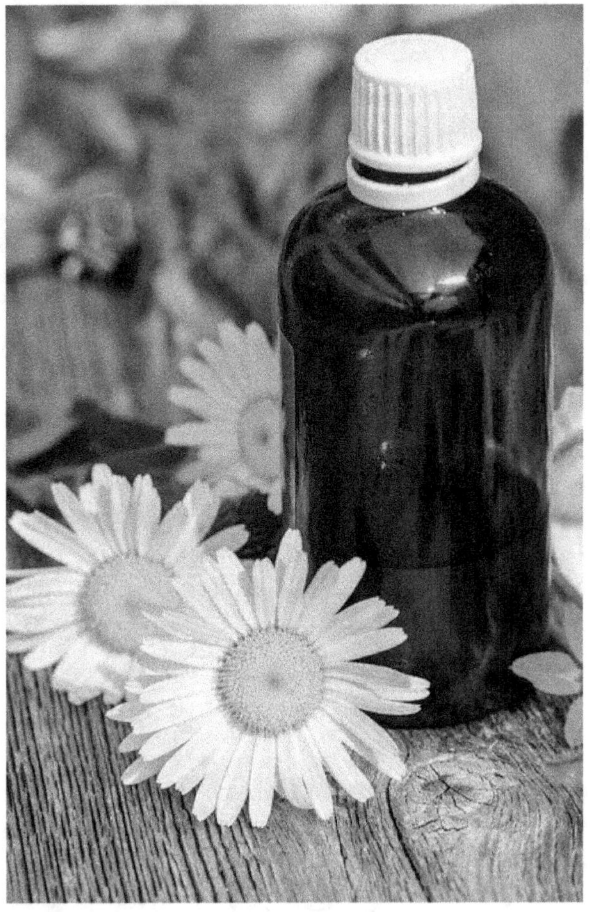

Fragrance Oils for Home Décor: Enhancing Your Living Space with Scent

References

Sources for further reading and research on fragrance oils and home décor

Sources for Further Reading and Research on Fragrance Oils and Home Décor

If you are interested in learning more about fragrance oils and how to use them in your home décor, there are many resources available to you. Whether you are a beginner or an experienced user of essential and fragrance oils, there is always something new to discover. Here are some sources for further reading and research on fragrance oils and home décor:

Books

There are many books available on the topic of fragrance oils and their use in home décor. Some of the most popular titles include "The Complete Book of Essential Oils and Aromatherapy" by Valerie Ann Worwood, "The Healing Art of Essential Oils" by Kac Young, and "The Fragrant Mind" by Valerie Ann Worwood.

Fragrance Oils for Home Décor: Enhancing Your Living Space with Scent

These books offer a wealth of information on the properties, uses and benefits of different essential and fragrance oils, as well as tips and techniques for incorporating them into your home décor.

Websites

There are many websites that provide information on fragrance oils and their use in home décor. Some of the best ones include AromaWeb, Essential Oil Haven, and The Spruce. These websites offer a wealth of information on the properties and uses of different essential and fragrance oils, as well as tips and techniques for incorporating them into your home décor. They also offer product reviews, recipes, and other helpful resources for those interested in exploring the world of fragrance oils.

Blogs

Blogs are a great source of information and inspiration for those interested in fragrance oils and home décor. Some of the most popular blogs on the topic include Aromatherapy School, The Essential Oil Company, and The Aromahead Blog.

These blogs offer a wealth of information on the properties and uses of different essential and fragrance oils, as well as tips and techniques for incorporating them into your home décor.

Fragrance Oils for Home Décor: Enhancing Your Living Space with Scent

They also offer product reviews, recipes, and other helpful resources for those interested in exploring the world of fragrance oils.

Conclusion

Whether you are a beginner or an experienced user of essential and fragrance oils, there are many resources available to you for further reading and research. From books to websites to blogs, there is always something new to discover about the properties, uses, and benefits of different fragrance oils and how they can enhance your home décor. So, take the time to explore these resources and discover the many ways in which fragrance oils can enhance your living space with scent.

www.ingramcontent.com/pod-product-compliance
Lightning Source LLC
Chambersburg PA
CBHW051831250726
48659CB00005B/1783